It's Not Just Stress

III

It's Not Just Stress: Recognizing Depression

Lesli Kramer, M.D.

SYREN BOOK COMPANY
Saint Paul

Published by
Syren Book Company LLC
2402 University Avenue West
Saint Paul, Minnesota 55114

Cover design: Kyle G. Hunter
Cover photo: Lesli Kramer

Printed in the United States of America on acid-free paper.

ISBN 0-929636-22-8

LCCN 2004102299

To order additional copies of this book see the order form at the back of the book or Amazon.com

*This is dedicated to my patients,
who provide a daily reminder
of the remarkable resiliency
of the human spirit,
and to each person who has said,
"I wish I would have known
about this a long time ago."*

Foreword

Do you have difficulty with unexplained aches and pains, fatigue, insomnia, or excessive need for sleep? Are you troubled by forgetfulness or loss of concentration? Do you experience persistent sadness, nervousness, frequent worrying, impatience, or loss of interest or pleasure in normal activities?

Have you wondered if you have depression or do you know someone with depression and want to understand what he or she is going through?

If so, this book can provide a glimpse that goes beyond standard symptom checklists, describing in detail the manner in which depressive symptoms manifest themselves in daily life. Many people, unaware that depression is more than a depressed mood, do not even consider the possibility that the problems they are experiencing are part of a depressive episode. Even when a person has been given a diagnosis of depression, they may not realize that certain problems, such as difficulty with concentration and memory, can be symptoms of depression.

It is my hope that this book will help people recognize depression. This initial recognition is a key to obtaining knowledge and appropriate treatment. It can be a great relief for a person with depression to finally have an explanation for why they feel so bad and to find out that they can feel better. My intent is to convey a message of hope and reassurance, and to help spread the word that depression is common, is not anyone's fault, and that it *can* get better.

This book can provide validation for people who have depression, whether or not it has been diagnosed. Many people experience similar kinds of symptoms, and seeing them in print can help people realize that they are not alone.

Because recognition, rather than treatment, is the major emphasis of this book, the scope is limited to a broad overview of possible symptoms and basic comments about depression. If you read this book and discover that you want to learn more, many fine books are available that provide comprehensive details about depression. A list of additional sources has been included at the end of this book.

The book is laid out in an easy-to-scan format, making it possible to learn some basic information about depression without delving into extended text.

No book can diagnose a depressive disorder, but if the experiences described in this book strike a chord of familiarity, you or the person you are concerned about should consider seeing a doctor.

Introduction

Depression is a common and frequently debilitating illness that often goes unrecognized and untreated. It is costly in terms of its impact on individuals, families, the workplace, and society in general. Unfortunately, only about one-third of people with depression seek help. The symptoms that comprise depression have been described since ancient times, but people no longer have to resign themselves to feeling miserable. We are fortunate to live in a time when there is finally hope for recovery.

One of the most important current challenges is educating people, since depression can only be treated if it is first recognized. Depression can be associated with physical symptoms that mimic other illnesses, and people frequently see their primary-care doctor for evaluation. Depression can be difficult to recognize and it doesn't always fit the expectations people have about how it looks or feels.

Depression is a brain disorder, an imbalance of brain chemicals. Anyone can develop depression, at any age. Hereditary factors play a role, and people are at increased risk of developing depression if it runs in their family. Stress can be a trigger, but depression can arise in the absence of stress, as well.

People often think that the depression is a temporary reaction, but even after the stress dissipates, the symptoms may not resolve because alterations in brain chemistry have occurred.

Depression can be severe or mild, of short duration or longstanding. Many symptoms of depression happen to everyone at some point in life. When trying to distinguish depression from "normal" experiences, a person must consider the frequency of these symptoms and the extent to which they impact daily life. Even mild depression, if it is ongoing or recurrent, can affect quality of life and interfere with a person's ability to live up to their full potential.

The stigma associated with depression sometimes prevents people from seeking treatment. In recent years, as more effective treatment options have become available, this barrier has been gradually eroding. As people are successfully treated, it becomes easier to recognize that depression is an actual medical disorder, not a personal weakness.

Depression is real. It is common. It is treatable.

A person can have many symptoms, or just a few. The following pages provide a glimpse of what it is like to live with depression.

It's Not Just Stress

///

People often don't know what's wrong. They feel overwhelmed and think it is "JUST STRESS."

Maybe it is. But it might be depression. People are sometimes surprised when it feels "so physical."

It is.

❚ Sleep can be a real problem.

Even if you are very tired, you may not sleep well at night. You might sleep for a few hours then wake up and toss and turn. Bleak hours may be spent awake, watching the clock, counting down the remaining hours left available to sleep. If you fall back to sleep, it seems as if you finally drop off into a good sleep just when it's time to wake up. You may have bad dreams, wake up feeling panicky, or not seem to dream at all anymore. You may sleep too much, for hours on end.

❚ It's difficult to "turn off your mind" to fall asleep.

You focus on a problem, some event that happened, or something you said or did. Your thoughts whirl around and around in your brain but you don't get anywhere. You can't seem to stop them.

❚ You are worn out, exhausted, and drained.

You don't feel refreshed, even if you've slept all night. Getting out of bed can be a struggle. You wake up and wonder how you will make it through the day.

▎ Your appetite may have changed.

You're not hungry, you forget to eat, food isn't appealing and you force yourself to eat. The thought of food makes you feel sick. Or, you may feel hungry all the time. You may eat to try to feel better, but the comfort from eating doesn't last very long.

▎ Preparing a meal is not on your agenda.

You grab something that's easy to eat. You may crave junk food or eat more carbohydrates and sweets.

▎ Your stomach is in a knot. You feel sick.

You may have headaches, a band-like pressure around your head, stomachaches, diarrhea, constipation, chest tightness, a choking sensation, a lump in your throat, and muscle aches and pains. Jittery feelings or a sense of internal shakiness can occur.

▎ Your mind can't relax. Your body can't relax.

It feels like adrenaline is coursing through your body. You feel "wired" and electrified.

▎ You can have many other physical symptoms.

It is possible to have sudden panic attacks with shortness of breath, heart racing, dizziness, shakiness, sweats, and feeling sick to your stomach. You might think you're going to faint. You may have chest pains and worry that you're having a heart attack.

▎ It's an effort to talk yourself into doing things.

Even small activities seem like a chore. Sometimes it's hard to get out of bed, shower, brush your teeth, or get dressed. You may stay in your pajamas all day. It seems like you can't get motivated or stay on top of your daily chores.

▎ Everything seems like hard work.

You feel weighted down, slow, and immobilized. You have to push yourself to get going. Your initiative is gone. Everything is a struggle.

▌ You procrastinate.

Small tasks, big tasks, it all seems overwhelming. You have to force yourself to get anything done. You postpone doing things, or don't do them at all and then feel guilty.

▌ Getting started can be the biggest problem.

It's like your spark plugs are malfunctioning. The part of your brain that initiates your "get up and go" may not be working right. Once you've gotten yourself moving, it is often easier to keep going. Like trying to get a boulder rolling downhill, getting started is the difficult part.

▌ Instead of feeling lethargic or slowed down, some people feel anxious and filled with nervous tension.

You may not be anxious *about* something, but feel wound up and on edge. It is a very "physical" feeling. Your body feels restless and it may be hard to sit still. You keep jumping up to do things. You can't sit through a movie or television show. It's hard to settle down. You may feel like you're going to jump out of your skin. Noises might bother you. You startle easily.

**｜ You may feel driven
to get things done.**

It seems like you can't possibly get all of your
work done. No sooner do you get started on one
thing than you think of something else that needs
to be done. It takes longer to accomplish things
because you jump from task to task.

**｜ You are overwhelmed.
Things feel out of control.**

It feels like you are under too much pressure. You
feel stressed. You may be hanging on by your finger-
nails. It is hard to cope and you don't think you
can handle much more. You are afraid that you are
falling apart.

｜ Your mind is preoccupied.

Your mind seems overly busy. You dwell on things
more than usual. It is hard to have thoughts of
anything other than your problems.

**▌ It's hard to feel at peace.
You worry about everything.**

You worry about the future and automatically
jump to negative conclusions. You worry about
bad things happening to people you care about. Old
problems resurface in your mind, even if you have
not thought about them for years. They suddenly
seem as difficult as when they were brand new.
Things that didn't seem to concern you previously
now bother you. The weight of the world rests on
your shoulders.

▌ You may be consumed by guilt.

You feel bad about things that have happened,
even if they occurred a long time ago. You are
filled with remorse. You mull over past errors and
criticize yourself harshly. You may find fault with
yourself for things that other people wouldn't give
a second thought to. Realistically, you may know
that you shouldn't feel guilty, but you have those
feelings anyway.

▌Some people find it hard to be alone.

You may be fearful or uncomfortable in situations that didn't bother you previously. Your anxiety gets the best of you. You need repeated assurances.

▌Being around other people can also be difficult.

You feel nervous and insecure. You don't feel like yourself. It's hard to think of anything to say. You worry that people will notice that you're having difficulty. Depression and anxiety drive a wedge between you and other people. You aren't able to connect. Even when you are with other people, you may feel very alone, possibly even more alone, because you feel so different. You over-analyze events and interactions with other people. You may be overly sensitive to actions or comments you perceive as rejection or criticism. You wonder what others are thinking of you, feel self-conscious, and assume the worst.

▌ Your self-confidence seems shattered.

You feel badly about yourself even if there is no reason: worthless, inadequate, and inferior, like a failure. You judge yourself more harshly than anyone else would. You are filled with self-doubt. You don't give yourself credit for your efforts or acknowledge your accomplishments.

▌ You withdraw.

The phone rings but you don't want to answer it. You let the answering machine get it. You don't return phone calls. You want to hide, pull the covers up over your head. You isolate yourself.

▌ Small things irritate you more than they should. You feel impatient.

Everything is magnified. You feel angry for no reason. You can't seem to let things roll off your shoulders; it is hard to take things in stride. Even things that normally would not be a problem can be blown out of proportion. You overreact and say things that you later regret. You are short-tempered, tense, crabby, and edgy. Your temper may flare when you are driving. Sometimes the least little thing makes you want to scream.

❚ You don't want to feel angry.
It just seems to happen.

You snap at people. You want people to leave you alone.

❚ A dark cloud comes over you.

It seems as if you've lost the ability to laugh. You try to force a smile. Things don't seem funny anymore. A wave of despair washes over you, a sense of doom and gloom is pervasive. You feel a sense of foreboding. The past, present, and future seem black. You feel like you are in a deep dark pit.

❚ You try to "put on a front."

You throw a wall up around yourself because you don't want others to know that you have depression.

❚ You act as if nothing is wrong.

You try to convince the world that everything is okay by putting on your "public face" and doing what you need to do to get through the day. Other people may think you would be the last person in the world to have depression because you can put on such a good front. It takes an extraordinary effort to maintain this facade, maybe all the strength you have. You get tired of pretending but you keep smiling anyway.

**| Not everyone can hide their
depression, at least not all of the time.**

It shows in your posture. Your limbs may feel
leaden. You may slump in your chair, walk slowly,
shuffle, avert your eyes, rest your head on your
hand, or sigh. People comment that you never
seem to smile. Your face appears drawn, lack-
ing your normal range of facial expression. Your
speech may be slowed down. You may speak
sharply to others, with an edge in your voice.

**| People ask you, "What's wrong?"
or, "Are you okay?"**

Even though you don't intend to look upset, your
face can appear sad or angry. You avoid eye con-
tact. Other people may think you are distant or
indifferent.

| You feel numb. Drained. Weary. Empty.

You may not feel happiness, sadness, anger, or
much of anything at all. There is a void, a hollow
feeling inside. Life may seem meaningless, everything is muted. You have a general feeling of heavi-
ness. It may seem like you don't have feelings for
other people anymore.

❚ You feel "sensitive."

You find yourself on the verge of tears for no particular reason. People ask you why you are crying but there isn't always an answer.

❚ You feel "negative."

If you have had depression for a long time, you may believe that your personality style tends toward pessimism. You assume that you are simply "a negative person." The cup seems half empty instead of half full. If something goes wrong, you have a tendency to think that *everything* is wrong.

❚ Things that once gave you pleasure no longer seem enjoyable.

Even if something good happens, you can't seem to feel better. You might have a brief glimmer of satisfaction, but then it's gone. Positive events don't sustain you like they should. Nothing seems like much fun.

▌ You don't look forward to anything anymore.

You avoid making any plans, in part because you're not certain you'll be up to doing anything when the time comes. You dread going anywhere and make excuses so you won't have to. It is hard to generate any enthusiasm, you feel like you are "going through the motions."

▌ Other people seem to experience happiness, and you wonder why the joy has gone out of *your* life.

Even things that should hold meaning for you do not seem to matter. Everything seems disappointing. Life feels futile.

▌ You feel apathetic.

You may not bother taking care of your appearance. You don't seem to care anymore. Nothing matters. Everything seems pointless.

▌ There is no luster.

Life seems dull, gray, flat, glum, bleak, dreary, and colorless: a dismal, gloomy void.

▌ You have lost interest in your normal activities.

Your friends, hobbies, or other interests don't have appeal. You may have lost all sexual desire. There is no spark. You may not even have realized how long it has been since you have done some of the things you used to enjoy. You don't want to go anywhere or do anything. It is hard to think of anything you might *want* to do. When you do go out, you can't wait to get back home.

▌ A sense of dread greets you in the morning. It takes all of your energy to make it through the day.

You can't wait until the day is over. You may go home and collapse. Tomorrow you manage to get up and do it again. You can't wait for the weekend, but when it arrives you still feel bad.

❙ You try to lose yourself in some activity, to escape for a while.

Shopping, eating, television, computer games, reading, gambling, and the Internet are all common escapes. You may stay up very late to have some quiet time for yourself or as a distraction so that you don't have to think. You may use drugs or alcohol to numb the pain or calm down, to try to feel "normal." You may retreat to bed and use sleep as an escape. You may pull the covers over your head and stay in bed all weekend.

❙ You may be forgetful.

You find yourself writing more notes. You can't remember what people have said to you. You repeat yourself in conversation. You make a phone call but can't remember whom you are calling. You miss appointments.

❙ You misplace things.

You can't find your keys, your glasses, your coffee cup, something you just had in your hand or your car in the parking lot.

▌ You feel disorganized.

You leave the house, but have to run back in repeatedly because you have forgotten something. You walk into a room but can't remember why you went there. You run up and down stairs because you forgot what you were going to do. You seem to be constantly behind schedule, running late. Everything feels chaotic.

▌ You have trouble recalling things that are well known to you.

If you are "put on the spot," it may be difficult to recall your birth date, your phone number, your social security number, or names of people you know well. That information is still in your brain, but it takes a while to access it.

▌ You search your brain for a word but "draw a blank."

You use the wrong word in a sentence and feel less articulate, at a loss for words. It's hard to convey your thoughts; it feels like there is a block. You lose track of what you are saying in mid-sentence and your speech is filled with pauses. You hesitate because you can't express yourself. You might misspell words, even words you used to be able to spell. Trying to write is a chore. Words do not flow.

▌ Everyday decisions seem difficult.

You struggle trying to decide what to wear, what to fix for dinner, what to buy at the grocery store, which restaurant to go to or what to order from the menu. You would rather have someone else decide. You don't have any strong preferences.

▌ It's hard to think.

Your thought processes feel dull, fragmented, and muddled. Your problem-solving ability is impaired. It is hard to generate ideas. You can't prioritize tasks. Balancing your checkbook is difficult. You make mistakes at work.

**| Time passes during the day and you
don't know where it all went.**

You shuffle through papers but don't really get
much done. You feel lost and don't know where
to start. You find yourself wandering aimlessly
around the house. It's hard to start projects and fin-
ish them. You lose track of time and "space out."

**| You jump from task to task
without completing anything.**

You can't get your work done in the normal
amount of time. One hour slips into the next.

**| You feel scattered.
Your mind wanders.**

You can't concentrate. Someone may be talking to
you, then you realize that you aren't paying attention. Nothing registers. It's frustrating.

| Reading can be difficult.

Your eyes scan the words but you don't have a clue
about what you have just read. You end up re-reading
sentences. Things just don't sink in. You may have
lost interest in reading simply because you can't.

▍ Driving may be a problem.

You might miss your freeway exit, leave your headlights on, lock your keys in the car, forget where you are going, or realize that you're not paying close attention to the road. You may back up your car or change lanes without checking to make sure that it is safe.

▍ You catch yourself staring into space.

You feel like you're in a fog. You may be preoccupied with your problems or simply devoid of thoughts, staring blankly.

▍ You may think you have attention deficit disorder.

Most people do not realize that depression can cause significant problems with concentration and memory. Treating the depression can improve these symptoms.

**❙ You worry that you have
  Alzheimer's disease.**

You might believe that your memory problems
are simply age related. While it is true that people
have some memory difficulty as a normal part of
aging, if you are having problems that seem trouble-
some, you should talk to a doctor. There are many
treatable illnesses that can interfere with memory,
including depression.

**❙ You fear that you have a terrible
  illness. Depression *is* terrible.**

The physical components of the illness can over-
shadow the emotional components. A person wor-
ried about their physical condition may think that
feeling down is just a natural consequence of their
worrying, rather than recognizing that the physical and emotional symptoms are all a part of one
illness: depression.

❚ You may think that if you were "a better person," you would not feel this way.

You might believe you've done something wrong, that you are being punished. You berate yourself and think that you are weak, stupid, lazy, selfish, sinful, or somehow defective. You try to convince yourself that if you simply tried harder, did more for other people, or quit focusing on yourself, you wouldn't be in this situation. You find fault with yourself and feel like you are no good. That's not true, but still you have those thoughts.

❚ You worry that you'll never get back to feeling like yourself again.

You are desperate to get better. It seems like a downward spiral. If you could depend upon getting relief at some point, it might be easier to bear, but depression often feels relentless. You pray tomorrow will be different, only to have that hope dashed. Hopelessness can set in. You may be at the point of giving up.

❚ You may wonder, "What's the point?" You may ask, "Why am I here?" and think that life is not worth living.

Those kinds of thoughts are not unusual for people experiencing depression. You think that if you got a serious illness, like cancer, you would not want to treat it, that it would be a blessing. It may seem like it would be easier if you were dead or just didn't wake up in the morning. Suicide may seem like a way out. You can't stand the thought of feeling this way day after day, year after year.

Most people don't end up acting on suicidal thoughts, but you have to take them seriously. Depression can be fatal, especially when it isn't recognized or treated. Even if you don't think you would act on them, suicidal thoughts are a signal that you should seek treatment.

You can feel better. That may seem hard to imagine right now, but you *can* recover.

Give yourself a chance. If you feel at risk for acting on suicidal thoughts call someone close to you, call a doctor, go to an emergency room, or call 911.

Depression is an inadequate name for this illness.
Depression isn't just having a bad day. It can be difficult to appreciate the painful depths that people experience when depression is severe. Depression can turn the world upside down. Feelings of self-esteem, competence, and self-assurance can be lost. Life feels bereft of joy or hope.

Depression is a misleading term. Everyone feels down or "depressed" at times, and people often do not realize that depression is more than feeling sad. Many people are unfamiliar with the spectrum of symptoms caused by depression, many of which have nothing to do with mood.

You can have "depression" and not even really "feel" depressed. People sometimes think depression always involves extreme sadness, constant crying, or inability to function, but in reality, many people are not affected to such a severe degree. Your mood may just be flat or "blah." You're not excited about much. Sometimes the very earliest symptoms are irritability, sleep problems, nervousness, fatigue, or concentration problems.

Depression has many faces. You can have many symptoms, or just a few. It doesn't look exactly the same in every person or at various points in time. Everyone is different.

People can have a low level of depression present for their entire life and not realize they have it. If depression is all you have ever known, you just live with it. You put one foot in front of the other and don't know that you can feel better. You may not even recognize that you've always had mild depression until you experience a more severe episode, seek treatment, and then begin to feel better, perhaps more consistently good than you can ever remember feeling before.

Depression can be *insidious*, creeping up slowly, infiltrating your life. You don't realize how bad it is until it feels as if you've run into a wall. You didn't see the depression developing, but in hindsight, it may have been coming on for a long time.

Even "mild" depression can affect the quality of a person's life, leading to a drab existence, devoid of joy, day after day. Even if life isn't totally without joy, depression can have an impact. Depression can influence choices and decisions that you make along the way. You may be experiencing problems on the job, at home, and in your relationships with people.

Many people think that if they moved, changed jobs, or left a relationship they would feel fine again. Maybe these are things that do need to be changed, but often depression colors the world a darker shade and affects the way you perceive and react to things. Making big changes while experiencing depression can also increase stress levels and cause a worsening of symptoms. It is often wise to postpone major decisions until your depression has lifted.

Some things may look different to you once the depression has cleared. Issues that you thought were important may disappear. You realize that they were a product of the depression. You may also recognize that there are other issues that *do* need to be addressed, issues that you couldn't see clearly until the depression got better.

People sometimes think it's "normal" to feel depressed when bad things have happened. It is normal to feel down when stressful events have occurred, but if you have developed *depression*, it means the stress has affected you physically. If you feel stuck, and it's not getting better, you should see a doctor.

People sometimes think that "when things get better" depression will go away by itself. Unfortunately, if you have depression, it doesn't necessarily lift when the stress has passed. If you developed a flat tire by running over a nail, your tire wouldn't automatically re-inflate when the nail was removed. Some action needs to be taken. Likewise, some action may need to take place for depression to improve, even when stress has been alleviated.

You may worry that other people will think that it's "all in your head" but you certainly *are not* imagining feeling this bad.

Depression is a real illness. Depression causes all sorts of physical symptoms in addition to the changes in your mood. The pain and discomfort are real. It feels like a physical illness because it *is* a physical illness. The primary problem is a change in the balance of your brain chemistry, which can then have a profound effect on your bodily functioning, thought processes, and emotions.

If there were any way to just snap out of it, you surely would have done just that. You may have thought that you should just pull yourself together. As more people are treated and realize that they don't have to feel so bad, it becomes easier for them to recognize that this is truly an illness. There is no reason to feel ashamed about having depression.

People often hope that there is some *other* medical explanation to account for their symptoms. For a lot of people, the symptoms seem more acceptable if they occur in the context of some other illness. Rest assured, however, that this is a real medical disorder.

Depression can just come out of the blue. Most people think that there has to be a reason to be depressed. There is often a connection to life events, but *not always*. People naturally try to link depression to something going on in their lives, but sometimes there is no external cause.

Although depression can "just happen," it can also be triggered by stress. If you already have depression, stressful events can make it worse. "Stress" can affect your brain chemistry and bodily functions. Your internal balance can be thrown off by a single stressful event or chronic ongoing stress, major problems, or a series of relatively minor stressors. Sometimes even *good* stress can trigger depression. Promotions, a new job, a move into a nice home—all may have been sought-after changes, but they *are* changes. Any shift in life circumstances can be stressful. Sometimes people manage to operate in crisis mode during a major event, and then feel like they fall apart afterwards. Even rock-solid seemingly unflappable people can be affected. Our bodies are not infallible. If you have a hereditary risk for developing depression, emotional or physical stress can be a trigger. Once you have had a depression triggered, you may be more prone to having it continue or develop again in the future, even without any stress.

Depression *is not about who you are*. It does not define you as a human being. You may be a person with depression but that does not mean you are a "depressed person."

You certainly are not alone. There is a good chance that you know a fair number of people who have depression. You might not be aware that they have it because people may not look or act depressed. Over the course of a lifetime, depression may affect up to twenty-five percent of the population.

Depression knows no boundaries. Anyone, from any walk of life, can develop depression; your neighbor, your best friend, the gas station attendant, teachers, lawyers, doctors, even presidents, like Abraham Lincoln. *Anyone can develop depression.*

No one is absolutely immune. It can happen to anyone, at any age: kids, teenagers, and adults, the very young to the very old. Sometimes people are just born with it. Depression could run in your family, though you may not know about it. People often don't talk about depression.

Depression can look different, depending on a persons age, gender, and individual biological make-up. There are some special considerations for people on either end of the age continuum.

Depression is common among older people. It's not just a normal part of aging. People tend to accumulate more losses as they age: occupations, friends, loved ones, health. It is not uncommon for depression to be overlooked in the face of all the losses. Older people sometimes complain of physical problems more than emotional symptoms. They may have prominent memory problems that lead people to believe they have Alzheimer's disease. Many people have been put in nursing homes when what they really needed was treatment for depression. It *is* possible to have both depression and dementia, in which case treating the depression may improve a person's ability to function.

Teenagers with depression may withdraw, isolate, seem bored and moody, become more argumentative or display open rebellion. It can be difficult to judge what is normal, but if they suddenly start performing poorly at school, it may not be "laziness." The concentration problems that occur as a result of depression can be misdiagnosed as attention deficit disorder. Teenagers may try to lose themselves in computer or video games. If an adolescent withdraws from friends, it's time to take notice. Normally, teenagers' sleep patterns include staying up later at night and waking up later. However, if a teenager seems tired all the time, sleeps too much, or cannot sleep well, there may be a problem.

Children with depression may complain about feeling sad, but often their depression is expressed in physical symptoms. Stomach aches and headaches are common. They may develop behavioral problems, seeming irritable and oppositional. They may withdraw from their friends, have difficulty getting along with other children, seem bored or unable to have fun. School performance may suffer because of problems with concentration, memory, and motivation. Again, it is not unusual for these children to be identified as having attention deficit disorder.

Depression can wax and wane according to the season or time of day. Some people have "seasonal" depression and feel much worse when the length of daylight decreases. Some people have "diurnal variation," which means that they have different levels of depression depending on the time of day. A common pattern is to feel terrible in the morning, with improvement as the day progresses. People may stay up late at night because that is when they finally feel decent. Our bodies have internal rhythms that are influenced by light / dark cycles, and depression can throw the natural balance out of synch.

Some other conditions increase vulnerability to depression. Multiple sclerosis, cancer, strokes, dementia, Parkinson's disease, heart disease, and other illnesses can predispose a person to depression, and the depression that develops is not just a psychological reaction to having a bad illness. The other illness may have upset the balance of your brain chemistry. Some medications, drugs, and alcohol can produce depressive symptoms, and they must be eliminated in order for the depression to remit. Girls and women who already have depression can feel much worse before their menstrual period. Postpartum hormonal changes can trigger depression, especially in women with a history of a previous episode or depression in their family. Depression is a very common illness and it is currently believed to be about twice as common in women.

Depression may worsen other illnesses or impair the recovery process. There can be a relationship between the presence of depression and recovery from a variety of illnesses, such as fibromyalgia, migraine headaches, and heart attacks. Treating the depression may improve your overall health and recovery.

Some illnesses may first manifest themselves with depressive symptoms. Problems such as thyroid disease, infectious mononucleosis, and nutritional deficiencies, among others, can be associated with symptoms that mimic depression. A clinical depression is the most common reason for depressive symptoms, but a doctor can discuss your symptoms with you and determine if you should be screened for any other illness.

Depression can affect every aspect of your being. In a physical sense, you may feel quite ill. On an emotional level, your sense of self may have been shaken to the very core. The thing that you may fear the most is never feeling like yourself again. But, with treatment, you *can* feel like yourself again.

Few illnesses make people feel so horrible, desperate, and hopeless that they might seriously consider killing themselves. Many people who have had other serious illnesses report that going through depression was more difficult.

Few illnesses steal away the capacity to experience joy. A beautiful day, a child's sunny smile, time spent with friends; during a depression, you may not be able to feel anything.

Nonetheless, there *is* hope. Depression can get better.

Wouldn't it be great to wake up one day and feel good? To feel a little spark of joy? To look forward to the day?

It can be normal to have some depressive symptoms on occasion but if you have frequent or persistent symptoms, or if they are adversely affecting your life, please don't dismiss them. Some days may not be so bad and that can really fool you. You might tell yourself that the depression is getting better, but if you step back and look at the big picture, you see a pattern of a lot of bad days and infrequent good days.

Depression still isn't talked about as freely as other illnesses, such as high blood pressure, diabetes, or cancer. But that is changing. The feelings of shame that burden people are lifted as more people realize that depression is a treatable illness and *not* a personality problem or character defect. When people who have been successfully treated for depression share their experience, other people often find it easier to seriously contemplate being evaluated and treated for depression.

One of the biggest hurdles to overcome may be acknowledging that you have depression. Fear of being labeled as "mentally ill" has been one of the greatest barriers to treatment. There remain a lot of misconceptions about depression, but as public awareness has grown, the stigma attached to the diagnosis has lessened.

Depression *is* very treatable. It can be a huge relief to find out that something can be done to help you feel better. You can feel like yourself again. You might just need a little help. Even if you have had chronic lifelong depression, you can feel better. There *is* effective treatment.

Depression isn't a sign of being weak. Neither is seeking help.

You wouldn't hesitate to seek help if you knew you were having a heart attack. Well, depression is also a medical problem.

Convincing yourself to go in for an evaluation can be difficult. Seeking treatment for the first time may not be easy, but once you've taken a step toward taking care of yourself, it gets easier. Seeing a psychiatrist does not mean that you are crazy. You are just one of many people who feel lousy because they have depression. Your family doctor or internist can often help. Call them.

You might not feel very strong, but consider the strength it takes to put one foot in front of the other when you feel so bad.

You can take that next step. You can talk to someone. You can see a doctor. You can discuss your symptoms. You *can* feel better.

Recommended Reading

Ainsworth, Patricia, M.D. 2000. *Understanding Depression.* Jackson: University Press of Mississippi.

DePaulo, J. Raymond, Jr., M.D., and Leslie Alan Horvitz. 2002. *Understanding Depression.* Hoboken, N.J.: John Wiley & Sons.

Gilbert, Paul. 2001. *Overcoming Depression.* New York: Oxford University Press.

Medina, John, Ph.D. 1998. *Depression: How it Happens, How it's Healed.* Hong Kong: New Harbinger Publications.

Papolos, Demitri, M.D., and Janice Papolos. 1997. *Overcoming Depression.* New York: HarperCollins.

Rosen, Laura Epstein, Ph.D., and Xavier Francisco Amador, Ph.D. 1997. *When Someone You Love Is Depressed.* New York: Simon & Schuster, Inc.

Resources

American Psychiatric Association
1400 K St. N.W.
Washington, DC 20005
(202) 682-6850
Web Site: www.psych.org

American Psychological Association
750 First St. N.E.
Washington, DC 20002-4242
(800) 374-2721
(202) 336-5510
TDD/TTY: (202) 336-6123
Web Site: www.apa.org

National Institute of Mental Health (NIMH)
Public Inquiries
6001 Executive Blvd., Room 8184, MSC 9663
Bethesda, MD 20892-9663
(301) 443-4513
TTY: (301) 443-8431
Fax: (301) 443-4279
Web Site: www.nimh.nih.gov

Depression Awareness, Recognition and Treatment (D/ART)
National Institute of Mental Health
5600 Fishers Lane
Rockville, MD 20857
(800) 421-4211

National Alliance for the Mentally Ill (NAMI)
2107 Wilson Blvd., Suite 300
Arlington, VA 22201
(703) 524-7600
(800) 950-NAMI (6264)
Fax: (703) 524-9094
Web Site: www.nami.org

National Mental Health Association
1021 Prince Street
Alexandria, VA 22314-2971
(703) 684-7722
Information Line (800) 969-NMHA (6642)
Fax: (703) 684-5968
Web Site: www.nmha.org

National Foundation for Depressive Illness
P.O. Box 2257
New York, NY 10116
(212) 268-4260 or (800) 239-1265
Fax: (212) 268-4434

Depression and Bipolar Support Alliance
730 North Franklin Street, Suite 501
Chicago, IL 60610-7224
(800) 826-3632
(312) 642-0049
Fax: (312) 642-7243
Web Site: www.DBSAlliance.org

Suicide Awareness Voices of Education (SA/VE)
7317 Cahill Road, Suite 207
Minneapolis, MN 55439-0507
(952) 946-7998 or 1-888-511-SAVE
Web Site: www.save.org

Acknowledgments

I am indebted to Matthew Collins for his thoughtful insights, suggestions, and reviews of this manuscript. Many thanks to Nora Collins, Lynne Dolan and Dr. Peggy Baker for their constructive commentary and encouragement. Special thanks go to the many people who have provided invaluable support, including Jane Schultz, R.N.—wonderful nurse, kindred spirit, dear friend. Jane Thompson, MSW, LICSW, BCD—ever irreverent friend with good shoes and a lot of letters after her name. Lou Bartholome, LP—terrific colleague and therapist. Debbra Ford, Psy.D.—smart, funny friend who plays a mean piano and is a darn good therapist. And Cheryl Karpen, my friend since childhood, with thanks for the strawberries, mud, and inspiration.

Lesli N. Kramer, M.D., is a graduate of the University of Minnesota Medical School. After completing her internship at the Hennepin County Medical Center in Minneapolis, MN, and her psychiatry residency at the University of Minnesota Medical School, she practiced psychiatry in a large multi-specialty group practice for ten years prior to entering her private practice in Eden Prairie, MN.

To order additional copies of *It's Not Just Stress:*

Web: www.itascabooks.com

Phone: 1-800-901-3480

Fax: Copy and fill out the form below with credit card information. Fax to 651-603-9263.

Mail: Copy and fill out the form below. Mail with check or credit card information to:

Syren Book Company
C/O BookMobile
2402 University Avenue West
Saint Paul, Minnesota 55114

Order Form

Copies	Title / Author	Price	Totals
	***It's Not Just Stress* / Kramer**	$8.95	$
		Subtotal	$
		7% sales tax (MN only)	$
		Shipping and handling, first copy	$ 4.00
		Shipping and handling, ___ add'l copies @$1.00 ea.	$
		TOTAL TO REMIT	$

Payment Information:

__ Check Enclosed __ Visa/Mastercard	
Card number:	Expiration date:
Name on card:	
Billing address:	
City:	State:	Zip:
Signature :	Date:

Shipping Information:

__ Same as billing address __ Other (enter below)	
Name:	
Address:	
City:	State:	Zip: